How to use POSTINOR

Your Guide to Safe and Effective Emergency Contraception

Natalie Callaway

Table of Contents

Introduction

Peace of Mind After Unprotected Sex

Life can be unpredictable. Sometimes, despite your best efforts, unexpected situations can arise, leaving you worried about the possibility of unwanted pregnancy. Postinor, an emergency contraceptive pill, can offer peace of mind in these moments.

This user guide is designed to provide you with clear and concise information about Postinor. We'll discuss what Postinor is, how it works, and when it might be the right option for you. We'll also address common concerns regarding its effectiveness, safety, and potential side effects.

Important Note: Postinor is not a substitute for regular birth control methods. It is intended for emergency use only. This guide will also explore the difference between emergency contraception and regular birth control methods, helping you choose the best approach for your overall sexual health.

By understanding your options and using this guide responsibly, you can make informed decisions about your reproductive health.

Chapter 1: Understanding Postinor

What is Postinor?

Postinor is an emergency contraceptive pill, often referred to as the "morning after pill." It's a safe and effective medication used to prevent pregnancy after unprotected sex or if your regular birth control method fails.

Postinor contains a synthetic hormone called levonorgestrel, which works differently than regular birth control pills. Regular birth control pills prevent ovulation (the release of an egg) or fertilization (the sperm meeting the egg). Postinor primarily works by delaying ovulation, but it may also impact the lining of your uterus, making it less hospitable for implantation if ovulation does occur.

When to Use Postinor

Postinor is most effective when taken as soon as possible after unprotected sex, ideally within 12 hours, but no later than 72 hours (3 days). The sooner you take Postinor, the higher its effectiveness.

Here are some situations where you might consider using Postinor:

You had unprotected sex and are not on any regular birth control.
Your condom broke or slipped off during sex.
Your diaphragm or cervical cap dislodged during sex.
You forgot to take one or more of your regular birth control pills according to the instructions.
You experienced sexual assault.

Important Note: Postinor is not effective if you are already pregnant. It will not terminate an existing pregnancy and will not

harm you or the fetus if you are already pregnant.

If you think you might be pregnant for reasons other than unprotected sex (e.g., missed period), Postinor is not the right option. In such cases, consult a doctor or healthcare provider for a pregnancy test and discuss your options.

Chapter 2: How Postinor Works and Important Information Before Use

How Postinor Works (Brief Overview)

While the exact mechanism of Postinor isn't fully understood, it's believed to work in two main ways, depending on where you are in your menstrual cycle:

Delaying Ovulation: If you haven't ovulated yet (released an egg), Postinor can prevent ovulation from happening by impacting hormones. This reduces the chance of an egg being available for fertilization by sperm.

Affecting the Uterine Lining: Even if ovulation has already occurred, Postinor may thicken the lining of your uterus, making it less receptive to a fertilized egg implanting.

Important Information Before Taking Postinor

Before using Postinor, it's essential to be aware of some important considerations:

Contraindications: While generally safe for most women, Postinor may not be suitable for everyone. If you have a history of blood clots, severe liver disease, undiagnosed vaginal bleeding, or are allergic to levonorgestrel or any other ingredients in Postinor, consult a doctor before taking it.

Potential Side Effects: Most women experience no serious side effects with Postinor. However, some common side effects include nausea, vomiting, fatigue, breast tenderness, headache, and dizziness. These side effects are usually mild and temporary.

Effectiveness: Postinor is most effective when taken within 12 hours of unprotected sex, with effectiveness decreasing the later it's taken. It's not 100% effective, and its success rate can be impacted by factors like your body weight.

Not Regular Birth Control: Postinor is for emergency use only and should not be used as a regular birth control method. It's best to discuss reliable birth control options with a doctor or healthcare provider.

Additional Considerations:

Interaction with Other Medications: Certain medications can interact with Postinor, potentially reducing its effectiveness. If you take other medications, consult a doctor or pharmacist to ensure there are no conflicts.

Pregnancy Test Not Required: A pregnancy test is not necessary before taking Postinor. However, if you experience a missed period after using Postinor, take a pregnancy test to rule out pregnancy.

Remember: This chapter provides a brief overview. It's crucial to read the information leaflet that comes with Postinor for complete details and instructions. If you have any concerns or questions, consult a doctor or healthcare professional before taking Postinor.

Chapter 3: Using Postinor Effectively

Taking Postinor correctly is essential for maximizing its effectiveness. This chapter will guide you through the proper dosage, timing, and administration of Postinor.

Dosage and Administration Instructions

Postinor comes in two variations:

Single Dose: This version contains one pill with a sufficient dose of levonorgestrel. Take the entire pill at once.

Two Dose: This version includes two pills. Take the first pill as soon as possible and the second pill exactly 12 hours later.

When to Take Postinor (Timeframe after Unprotected Sex)

The effectiveness of Postinor is highly time-dependent. Here's a breakdown:

Most Effective: Take the first dose (or single pill) within 12 hours of unprotected sex. The sooner you take it, the better the chance it will prevent pregnancy.

Effective: Take the first dose (or single pill) within 72 hours (3 days) of unprotected sex. While still effective, its success rate decreases the later it's taken.

Ineffective: Postinor will not work if you are already pregnant.

How to Take Postinor (With or Without Food)

Postinor can be taken with or without food. However, if you experience nausea or vomiting after taking it with food, you can take the second dose (if applicable) on an empty stomach or with a light snack.

Important Tips:

Read the Package Leaflet: Always refer to the information leaflet that comes with your specific version of Postinor for detailed instructions.

Follow the Timeframe: Taking Postinor outside the recommended time frame (72 hours) significantly reduces its effectiveness.

Don't Take More Than Needed: Taking more than the recommended dose will not increase effectiveness and may cause unnecessary side effects.

If you have any questions or are unsure about using Postinor, consult a doctor or healthcare professional for personalized guidance.

Chapter 4: Understanding Postinor's Effectiveness

While Postinor can be a valuable tool for preventing unwanted pregnancy after unprotected sex, it's important to understand its effectiveness and limitations.

How Effective is Postinor?

Postinor's effectiveness depends on when you take it:

Most Effective (Within 12 Hours): Studies suggest Postinor can prevent up to 95% of expected pregnancies when taken within the first 12 hours after unprotected sex.

Effective (Within 72 Hours): If taken within 72 hours (3 days) of unprotected sex, Postinor's effectiveness is estimated to be around 85%.

Ineffective (After 72 Hours): Postinor is not effective if taken more than 72 hours after unprotected sex.

Factors Affecting Effectiveness

Several factors can influence Postinor's effectiveness:

Timing: As mentioned above, the sooner you take Postinor, the more effective it will be.
Body Weight: Postinor may be less effective for women with a body mass index (BMI) exceeding 30.

Important Considerations:

Not Guaranteed: It's important to remember that Postinor is not 100% effective. Even if taken correctly, there's still a chance of pregnancy.
Not Regular Birth Control: Postinor is for emergency use only and should not be relied on as a primary method of birth control.

Understanding Your Risk:

If you're considering using Postinor, talk to a doctor or healthcare professional. They can help you assess your individual risk of pregnancy based on factors like your cycle and when you had unprotected sex. This can help you decide if Postinor is the right option for you.

Chapter 5: Safety and Side Effects of Postinor

Postinor is generally safe for most women, but like any medication, it can cause side effects. This chapter will outline the common side effects, potential for more serious reactions, and when to seek medical attention.

Common Side Effects of Postinor

Most women who take Postinor experience no serious side effects. However, some common side effects may occur, including:

Nausea and vomiting: These are the most common side effects and may occur within a few hours of taking Postinor.

Fatigue: You may feel tired or experience headaches after taking Postinor.

Breast tenderness: Some women experience breast tenderness or swelling after using Postinor.

Abdominal pain or cramping: Mild cramping or discomfort in the lower abdomen may occur.

Dizziness: You may experience slight dizziness after taking Postinor.

Spotting or irregular bleeding: Changes in your menstrual bleeding pattern are common after taking Postinor. Your next period may be earlier, later, heavier, or lighter than usual.

Less Common But More Serious Side Effects

While uncommon, some more serious side effects can occur with Postinor. Seek medical attention immediately if you experience:

Severe abdominal pain or cramping
Heavy vaginal bleeding that soaks through pads in an hour
Signs of an allergic reaction, such as swelling of the face, lips, tongue, or throat, difficulty breathing, or hives

When to Seek Medical Attention After Taking Postinor

If you experience any concerning side effects not listed above, consult a doctor or healthcare professional. Additionally, seek medical attention if:

You vomit repeatedly and cannot keep Postinor down.

You miss your expected period after using Postinor and taking a pregnancy test is negative. There's a small chance the pregnancy could be ectopic (located outside the uterus), which requires urgent medical attention.

You have concerns or questions about using Postinor.

This information is intended for general knowledge only. If you have any questions or experience any concerning side effects, consult a doctor or healthcare professional for personalized guidance.

Chapter 6: Postinor and Your Birth Control Regimen

Will Postinor Affect My Regular Birth Control?

Generally, Postinor will not interfere with your existing hormonal birth control methods (e.g., birth control pills, patch, or ring). However, there are a few things to consider:

Combined Oral Contraceptives (COCs): If you take COCs (birth control pills containing both estrogen and progestin), Postinor likely won't affect their effectiveness. You can continue taking your regular birth control pills as usual after using Postinor.

Progestin-Only Pills (POPs): If you take POPs (birth control pills containing only progestin), Postinor might slightly decrease their effectiveness. This is because both medications contain progestin, and the additional progestin from Postinor may interact with your regular pills. To be safe, consider using a backup method of contraception (e.g., condoms) for the next week after taking Postinor.

Important Note: If you have any concerns about how Postinor might interact with your specific birth control method, consult a doctor or pharmacist for personalized advice.

Using Postinor While on Other Medications

Certain medications can interact with Postinor, potentially reducing its effectiveness. Here's what to know:

Medications that Affect Hormone Breakdown: These medications, like certain antibiotics, antifungals, and anti-seizure medications, can accelerate the breakdown of hormones in your body, including the levonorgestrel in Postinor. This can make Postinor less effective.

St. John's Wort: This herbal supplement can also interact with Postinor, potentially reducing its effectiveness.

What to Do:

Inform Your Doctor or Pharmacist: Before using Postinor, tell your doctor or pharmacist about all the medications you currently take, including prescription drugs, over-the-counter medications, and herbal supplements.
Alternative Options: If you take medications that interact with Postinor, your doctor might recommend alternative emergency contraception methods, such as the copper IUD, which is not affected by other medications.

It's crucial to disclose all medications you take to ensure Postinor's effectiveness and avoid potential interactions.

Chapter 7: Emergency Contraception vs. Regular Birth Control: Understanding Your Options

Postinor is a valuable tool for preventing unwanted pregnancy after unprotected sex. However, it's not a substitute for regular birth control methods. This chapter explores the key differences between Postinor and regular birth control options, helping you choose the best approach for your needs.

Emergency Contraception (Postinor)

Function: Prevents pregnancy after unprotected sex by delaying ovulation or affecting the uterine lining.

Effectiveness: Effectiveness depends on timing, ranging from 85% to 95% when taken within 72 hours of unprotected sex.

Use: Intended for emergency use only, not a reliable long-term solution.

Side Effects: May cause nausea, vomiting, fatigue, breast tenderness, and irregular bleeding.

Availability: Available over-the-counter without a prescription in most places.

Regular Birth Control Methods

Function: Work in various ways to prevent pregnancy before sex, including preventing ovulation, blocking sperm from reaching the egg, or thickening cervical mucus.

Effectiveness: Highly effective (over 99% typical use) when used correctly.

Use: Intended for ongoing pregnancy prevention.

Side Effects: Varies depending on the method, but may include changes in bleeding patterns, breast tenderness, mood swings, and headaches. Some methods have minimal to no side effects.

Availability: Variety of methods available, some requiring a prescription from a doctor or healthcare provider. Options include:

Oral contraceptive pills (combined or progestin-only)

Vaginal ring

Patch

IUD (copper or hormonal)

Injections

Implants

Choosing the Right Option

Emergency Situations: If you've had unprotected sex and are concerned about pregnancy, Postinor can be a helpful option. However, it's most effective when taken as soon as possible.

Ongoing Protection: If you're sexually active and want reliable pregnancy prevention, regular birth control methods are the best choice. They offer much higher effectiveness and can be tailored to your individual needs and preferences.

Consulting a Doctor or Healthcare Provider

Discussing your birth control options with a doctor or healthcare provider is crucial. They can help you:

Choose the most suitable birth control method based on your health history, lifestyle, and preferences.
Address any concerns you have about Postinor or regular birth control methods.
Provide guidance on proper use of your chosen birth control method to maximize its effectiveness.

Both Postinor and regular birth control methods have their roles in preventing unwanted pregnancy. Understanding their differences empowers you to make informed choices about your sexual health.

Chapter 8: Additional Information about Postinor

Where to Get Postinor

Access to Postinor can vary depending on your location. Here are some common options:

Pharmacies: In many places, Postinor is available over-the-counter at pharmacies without a prescription. It's best to call your local pharmacy beforehand to confirm availability and pricing.

Family Planning Clinics: Family planning clinics often provide Postinor and other emergency contraception options. They may also offer additional services like pregnancy testing, STI testing, and counseling.

Online Retailers: Some reputable online retailers may sell Postinor, but exercising caution is essential. Ensure the retailer is licensed and offers legitimate products.

Cost of Postinor

The cost of Postinor can vary depending on the brand, pharmacy, or retailer.

Chapter 9: Understanding Postinor-2 Specifically

While the general information about Postinor applies to Postinor-2 as well, there are some specific details to consider regarding this particular brand version.

Dosage and Administration:

Postinor-2 comes in a single-dose format. This means there's only one pill to take, unlike some other emergency contraceptive brands that require two doses.

Take the single Postinor-2 pill as soon as possible after unprotected sex, ideally within 12 hours, but no later than 72 hours (3 days).

Following the same principles as with other Postinor variations:

The sooner you take Postinor-2, the more effective it will be.

Postinor-2 is not effective if you are already pregnant.

Benefits of a Single-Dose Option:

Simplicity: Having just one pill to take can be easier to remember and manage, especially in stressful situations.
Convenience: No need to worry about taking a second dose 12 hours later.

Important Considerations:

Read the Package Leaflet: Always refer to the information leaflet that comes with your specific Postinor-2 pack for detailed instructions.
Effectiveness: Even with the single-dose format, Postinor-2's effectiveness remains similar to other Postinor versions, ranging from 85% to 95% depending on when it's taken.

In conclusion, Postinor-2 offers a convenient and effective emergency contraceptive option with a single-dose format. Remember, for the best results, take it as soon as possible after unprotected sex. If you have any questions or concerns, consult a doctor or healthcare professional.

Appendix

Glossary of Terms

Emergency Contraception (EC): Medications used to prevent pregnancy after unprotected sex.

Ovulation: The release of an egg from the ovary.

Uterus: The muscular organ in a woman's body where a fetus develops during pregnancy.

Hormones: Chemical messengers produced by glands in the body that regulate various functions.

Levonorgestrel: The synthetic hormone present in Postinor that works to prevent pregnancy.

Menstrual Cycle: The monthly series of changes in a woman's body that prepares her for a potential pregnancy.

Body Mass Index (BMI): A measurement used to categorize weight-to-height ratio.

Ectopic Pregnancy: A pregnancy that develops outside the uterus, usually in the fallopian tubes.

St. John's Wort: An herbal supplement sometimes used for depression.

IUD (Intrauterine Device): A T-shaped device inserted into the uterus to prevent pregnancy.

Cervical Mucus: Mucus produced by the cervix that can thicken and block sperm during certain phases of the menstrual cycle.

Frequently Asked Questions (FAQs)

About Postinor:

Q: How long do I have to take Postinor after sex?

A: Postinor is most effective the sooner you take it, ideally within 12 hours of unprotected sex, but no later than 72 hours (3 days).

Q: Can I take Postinor if I'm already pregnant?

A: No. Postinor will not terminate an existing pregnancy and will not harm you or the fetus if you are already pregnant.

Q: Will Postinor affect my regular birth control?

A: Generally, no. However, consult your doctor or pharmacist if you have any concerns.

Q: Can I get Postinor over-the-counter?

A: Access to Postinor can vary by location. In many places, it's available over-the-counter without a prescription. It's best to check local guidelines.

Using Postinor:

Q: Do I need a prescription for Postinor?

A: It depends on your location. In many places, Postinor is available over-the-counter.

Q: Can I take Postinor with food?

A: Yes, you can take Postinor with or without food.

Q: What if I vomit after taking Postinor?

A: If you vomit within one hour of taking Postinor, contact a doctor or pharmacist for guidance. You may need to take another dose.

After Taking Postinor:

Q: Will Postinor affect my period?

A: You may experience some spotting or irregular bleeding after taking Postinor. Your next period may be earlier, later, heavier, or lighter than usual. If you miss your expected period and take a pregnancy test that is negative, consult a doctor to rule out ectopic pregnancy.

Q: Can I get pregnant again right away after using Postinor?

A: Yes. Postinor does not prevent ovulation in your next cycle. It's important to use a regular birth control method if you don't want to get pregnant.

Remember: This FAQ is not exhaustive. If you have any questions or concerns not addressed here, consult a doctor or healthcare professional.

9 798321 606209